NURSING MNEMONICS

100 + Memory Tricks to Crush the Nursing School
&
Trigger Your Nursing Memory

Maria Youtman
MSN BSN RN

When I think about all the patients and their loved ones that I have worked with over the years, I know most of them don't remember me nor I them. But I do know that I gave a little piece of myself to each of them and they to me and those threads make up the beautiful tapestry in my mind that is my career in nursing.

#Donna Wilk Cardillo

Contents

6

INTRODUCTION

There are a ton of terms that need to be read and memorized to help you at your nursing school, as well before you take the NCLEX-RN Exam.

It may get pretty hard to remember all of those concepts right off hand. One good way to help you to remember certain terms and concepts is to use Mnemonics.

Everyone has their own way of remembering information and that's why NCLEX-RN mnemonics are so helpful. Mnemonics is the study and development of systems for improving and assisting the memory.

Using mnemonics is an excellent way to keep things straight while also relating them to something less stressful.

Mnemonics improve your memory by using the technique of association.

At this Book, you get the most helpful mnemonics for the NCLEX-RN exam that you should include in your study sessions.

TERMINAL OBJECTIVES:

Mnemonics are popular study aids to help trigger your memory of a group of things. It is similar to memorizing a phone number. Instead of memorizing each individual number – you remember a group of 3 numerals (area code), 3 numbers and a group of 4 numbers. This is called "chunking". When one thinks of a mnemonic, you usually think of a list of vertical letters that spell a word with words going off the stem horizontally.

For example: What you should quickly do with an acute myocardial infarction (MI/heart attack)?
M – morphine sulfate
O – oxygen
N – nitroglycerine
A – ASA (acetylsalicyclic acid)

In this instance, remembering the word "**MONA**" = MI, can help you remember all the nursing actions one should anticipate.

Mnemonics are not always words however. They can really be any words, pictures, diagrams, lyrics/songs, a rhyme, or something that forms a relationship to help you remember.

Sometimes even the process of creating or thinking up a mnemonic can help you learn the underlying concept. My brain often likes to draw diagrams or models. Flowcharts or hierarchies can help me understand how things work together.

Personally, mnemonics to me have been helpful for some concepts but not all. I don't really learn well with tons of mnemonics; I just have a couple for things that are really hard for me to remember.

Sometimes it seems like it is just as much work to learn the mnemonic as it would be just to memorize the information.

That is why the actual process of trying to think of a drawing, picture, diagram, or acronym can actually be more useful than just using someone else's mnemonic.

Recognize The Following Example:

The American Cancer Society uses **"CAUTION"** to describe cancer warning signs:

C – change in bowel or bladder habits
A – a sore that does not heal
U – unusual bleeding or discharge
T – thickening or lump
I – indigestion or difficulty swallowing
O – obvious change in size of a wart or mole
N – nagging cough or hoarseness

What are depressant drugs?

"Bats" Barbiturates, Alcohol, and Tranquilizers

You can draw a picture of a limp bat to help you remember this one...

SOAP Note
S – Subjective
O – Objective
A – Assessment
P – Plan

There are even now some diagnoses that are acronyms/mnemonics. An example is "HELLP Syndrome" which stands for **H**emolysis, **E**levated **L**iver enzymes and **L**ow **P**latelets or **HELLP**. HELLP syndrome is a life-threatening obstetric complication considered to be a complication of pre-eclampsia. The only treatment is delivery of the baby.

Mnemonics can even be how you take notes. Most people think of notes as an outline where you try to scribble as fast as the teacher talks. However, you can take notes a couple of different ways that can help you remember the information, rather than writing down all the words.

- If your teachers provide printed outlines: then draw pictures or diagrams of what they are talking about in the margin. This helps you use both sides of your brain and associate concepts.

- You can fold 1/3 of your page vertically and make a crease. On the left side of the crease you can write a question that you think of while they are talking. This is called the cue column. Literally make the concept into a test question. On the right side of the crease - right the answers or key ideas. At the bottom of the page, summarize the whole idea or concept in your own sentence. Later when you look back through your notes to study, you can fold the paper and "hide" the answers from yourself. It is a lot easier to keep track of then notecards.

This is called the Cornell System of notetaking. You can usually even find notepaper formatted this way to make it easy in office supply stores.

Nursing Health Assessment Mnemonics

Level of Consciousness Assessment: "AVPU"

The AVPU scale is a system where you can measure and record a patient's responsiveness to indicate their level of consciousness. It is a simplification of the Glasgow Coma Scale, which assesses a patient response in three measures: eyes, voice, and motor skills. The AVPU scale should be assessed during these three identifiable traits, looking for the best response for each. It has four possible outcomes for recording and the nurse should always work from best (A) to worst (U) to avoid unnecessary tests on patients who are clearly conscious. On the other hand, it should not be used for long-term follow up of neurological status.

A	Alert
V	Response to Verbal Stimuli
P	Response to Pain
U	Unresponsive

Have you heard, "The patient is unconscious, breathing, and talking" and thought?"

The AVPU scale — a tool used to assess the patient's brain perfusion and function — describes a patient's level of consciousness.

A = the patient is **Awake**

V = the patient responds to a **Verbal** stimulus

P = the patient responds to a **Pain** stimulus
U = the patient is **Unresponsive** to stimulus

The distinction between 'A' and 'V' frequently causes confusion.
You are awake on AVPU scale

If you are reading this, you are 'A' on AVPU. You might be awake and confused, awake and disoriented, awake and lethargic, or awake and oriented.

Awake patients are always awake and some adjective that describes their mental status of being awake.
Not Awake is unconscious

A patient that is not awake is unconscious, V, P, or U.

A patient that is 'V' responds to a verbal stimulus provided by responders.

Have you ever yelled, "DUDE, wake up!" to an intoxicated patient (or friend) and they raised their eyes, looked at you, or somehow responded to your voice? They are responding to a verbal stimulus.

If the patient responds, "Why are you yelling at me?" the patient is 'A.'

A patient that is 'V' cannot be alert, answer history questions, or describe their chief complaint.
Interpreting a pain stimulus

If the patient doesn't respond to a verbal stimulus attempt a pain stimulus with a pinch, squeeze or sternum rub.

A sternum rub is the application of painful stimulus with the knuckles of closed fist to the center chest of a patient who is not alert and does not respond to verbal stimuli. The sternum rub is the most common painful stimulus practiced in the field by EMTs and paramedics. However, it is possible to misinterpret the patient's response to the stimuli depending on the duration the pressure is applied.

Health History Assessment: "SAMPLE"

In general, do not obtain a detailed history until life-threatening injuries have been identified and therapy has been initiated. The secondary survey is essentially a head-to-toe assessment of progress, vital signs, etc. SAMPLE is often useful as a mnemonic for remembering key elements of the patient's health history.

S	Symptoms
A	Allergy
M	Medications
P	Past Medical History
L	Last Oral Intake
E	Events leading up to the illness or injury

- **S: Symptoms: Patient chief complain.**
  Question to ask: what's wrong?
  What brought you to the hospital?

- **A: Allergy: Seeking to know what type of allergic reaction they experience.**
  Question to ask: Do you have allergy to anything?
  What happens to you when you use something you are allergic to?

- **M: Medications: Prescribed OTS drugs, herbal meds.**
  Question to ask: Are you taking any medication?
  What are you taking the medication for?
  When did you last take your medication?

- **P: Past Medical History: seeking to know the previous state of health, and previous illness.**
  Question to ask: Have you had this problem before?
  Do you have any other health problems?

- **L: Last Oral Intake: Seeking what are the last oral intakes of the patient.**
  Question to ask: When did you last eat or drink anything?
  What was it that last you intake?

- **E: Events leading up to the illness or injury.**
  Question to ask: How did you get hurt?
  What led to this problem?

Rapid Trauma Assessment: "DCAP-BTLS"

DCAP-BTLS is a mnemonic to remember specific soft tissue injuries to look for during assessment of a person after a traumatic injury.

D	Deformities
C	Contusions
A	Abrasions
P	Punctures or Penetrations
B	Burn
T	Tenderness
L	Lacerations
S	Swelling

D: Deformities
Malformations or distortions of the body.

C: Contusions
Injury to tissues with skin discoloration and without breakage of skin; also called a bruise.

A: Abrasions
Scrape caused by rubbing from a sharp object resulting in surface denuded of skin.

P: Punctures or Penetrations
Wound with relatively small opening compared with the depth; produced by a narrow pointed object.

B: Burns
Burns are injuries to tissues caused by heat, friction, electricity, radiation, or chemicals.

T: Tenderness
The condition of being tender or sore to the touch.

L: Lacerations
A torn or jagged wound caused by blunt trauma; incorrectly used when describing a cut.

S: Swelling
Sign of inflammation; caused by the exudation of fluid from the capillary vessels into the tissue.

Alcoholism Screening: "CAGE"

CAGE questionnaire is a widely used and an extensively validated method of screening for alcoholism. Two "yes" responses indicate that the possibility of alcoholism should be investigated further. By far the most important question in the CAGE questionnaire is the use of a drink as an Eye Opener, so much so that some clinicians use a "yes" to this question alone as a positive to the questionnaire; this is because the use of an alcoholic drink as an Eye Opener connotes dependence since the patient is going through possible withdrawal in the morning, hence the need for a drink as an Eye Opener.

C	CONCERN by the person that there is a problem
A	APPARENT to others that there is a problem
G	GRAVE consequences
E	EVIDENCE of dependence or tolerance

- **C:** Have you ever felt that you should **CUT** down on your drinking?
- **A:** Have you ever become **ANNOYED** by criticisms of your drinking?
- **G:** Have you ever felt **GUILTY** about your drinking?
- **E:** Have you ever had a morning **EYE OPENER** to get rid of a hangover?

Emergency Trauma Assessment: "ABCDEFGHI"

The **ABCDEFGHI** mnemonic is used for a quick assessment of trauma patients. This is especially useful for emergency cases. The purpose of primary assessment is to preserve the life of the victim, taking action where needed. Once the victim's life-threatening conditions have been address, the rescuer must begin secondary assessment.

Primary Survey	
A	Airway
B	Breathing
C	Circulation
Secondary Survey	
D	Disability
E	Expose & Examine
F	Full set of vital signs
G	Give comfort measures
H	History and Head-To-Toe Assessment
I	Inspect Posterior Surface

A: Airway
Keep the airway open to allow the body to take in oxygen and expel carbon dioxide. Use the head-tilt chin-lift technique to open the airway. Check or and remove obstructions. A blocked airway can lead to respiratory or cardiac arrest.

B: Breathing
Once the airway is open, check for normal breathing, make use of the look, listen, and feel techniques.
Look at the chest and observe the rising and falling for normal respiration. Listen for air movement. Feel for air coming through the mouth or nose. If there is no breathing or abnormal breathing, CPR must be initiated with 2 breaths.

C: Circulation
Oxygen-rich blood cannot be circulated without breathing. Hence, it's unnecessary to check for pulse to determine whether CPR is needed; commence immediately if no breathing is detected.

D: Disability
Check the patient's neurological status and for obvious deformities or disabilities.

E: Expose & Examine
Remove clothing to properly assess patient; be sure to keep the patient warm.

F: Full set of vital signs
Note any changes in the following signs: pulse (carotid, brachial, radial), pupils, breathing, level of consciousness, blood pressure, and skin color and temperature.

G: Give comfort measures
Continue to rest and reassure. Provide comfort measures and prevent further injury.

H: History and Head-To-Toe Assessment
Use the mnemonic SAMPLE to obtain health history and do a head-to-toe assessment after.

I: Inspect Posterior Surface
Inspect for wounds, deformities, discolorations, etc.

Seven Warning Signs of Cancer

"CAUTION"

Early detection is the key in treatment of cancers. The CAUTION mnemonic is used by the American Cancer Society to detect and recognize the early warning signs of cancer. Though one of these signs does not necessarily mean someone has cancer.

C	Change in bowel or bladder habits
A	A sore throat that does not heal
U	Unusual bleeding or discharge
T	Thickening or lump in breast or elsewhere
I	Indigestion or dysphagia
O	Obvious change in wart or mole
N	Nagging cough or hoarseness

- **C: Change in bowel or bladder habits**
  Common sign of colorectal cancer.

- **A: A sore throat that does not heal**
  If located on the skin or in the mouth, skin cancer or mouth cancer could be the cause.

- **U: Unusual bleeding or discharge**
  Any bleeding from the bladder, vagina or rectum could mean prostate, cervical or colorectal cancer.

- **T: Thickening or lump in breast or elsewhere.**
  A lump on the breast can be sign of cancer, a lump on the testicle can be testicular cancer.

- **I: Indigestion or dysphagia.**
  Can be symptoms of stomach, throat, esophagus or mouth cancer.

- **O: Obvious change in wart or mole.**
  Most common sign of skin cancer.

- **N: Nagging cough or hoarseness**
  A cough last for four weeks or longer can be symptoms of lung and/or throat cancer.

Family History Assessment

"BALD CHASM"

Family history plays a critical role in assessing the risk of inherited medical conditions, chronic illnesses and genetically transmitted diseases. Outline or diagram age and health, or age and cause of death of siblings, parents, and grandparents. Document presence or absence of specific illnesses in family. Use the mnemonic "BALD CHASM" to recall the diseases that needs to be investigated.

B	Blood pressure
A	Arthritis
L	Lung diseases
D	Diabetes
C	Cancers
H	Heart diseases
A	Alcoholism
S	Stroke
M	Mental health disorders

B: Blood pressure
African Americans have a higher risk for high blood pressure. Poor lifestyle choices and diet, that can be inherited by the family, can also pose as a risk.

A: Arthritis
Some types of arthritis run in families. Genes can be a contributing factor that can make someone susceptible to environmental factors that may trigger arthritis.

L: Lung diseases
Cystic fibrosis is a common inherited disease that affects mostly the lungs. It is manifested by accumulation of thick, sticky mucous, frequent infections and coughing.

D: Diabetes
History of type 2 diabetes in the family poses the patient at increased risk of developing it.

C: Cancers
Certain types of cancer, such as breast cancer and colon cancer, appear more frequently in some families.

H: Heart diseases
Genes can pass on the risk of cardiovascular disease, and they can also be responsible for passing on other conditions such as high blood pressure or high cholesterol levels.

A: Alcoholism
Certain genetic factors influence alcoholism. Research show that children of alcoholics are about four times more likely than the general population to develop alcohol problems.

S: Stroke
Risk for stroke is higher if someone in the patient's direct family line that stroke. Some strokes may be symptoms of genetic disorders like CADASIL.

M: Mental health disorders (depression, bipolar, schizophrenia etc.)
Some mental illnesses can run in families, although it may be from variety of factors rather than just genes.

Breast Assessment: "LMNOP"

Breast masses show marked variation in etiology, from fibro adenomas to cysts, to abscesses, mastitis, to breast cancer. All breast masses warrant careful evaluation, and definitive diagnostic measures should be pursued.

L	Lump
M	Mammary changes
N	Nipple changes
O	Other symptoms
P	Patient risk factors

L: Lump
Inspect and palpate breast for lumps, masses.

M: Mammary changes
Inspect and palpate for dimpling, tenderness, abnormal contours.

N: Nipple changes
Inspect and palpate for nipple retraction, lesions, discharges.

O: Other symptoms
Check size, symmetry, appearance of skin, direction of pointing, rashes, and ulceration.

P: Patient risk factors
Interview patient for predisposing factors, obtain family history or use the Breast Cancer Risk Assessment Tool.

Eyes Abbreviation

Abbreviations for the eyes are often confusing. OU which stands for the latin term Oculus Uterque means both eyes; OD for Oculus Dexter referring to the right eye and OS for Oculus Sinister for the left eye. Remember the mnemonic above to make sense of these abbreviations.

- **YOU** look with **BOTH** eyes.
- The **RIGHT** dose won't **OD** [overdose].
- The only one that is **LEFT** is **OS**.

Signs VS Symptoms

Signs are commonly distinguished from symptoms and both are something abnormal and relevant to a potential medical condition. A sign is objective and is discovered by the health-care professional during an examination whereas a symptom is subjective, observed and experienced by the patient, and cannot be measured directly.

- sIgn: something I can detect even if patient is unconscious.
- sYMptom is something only hYM knows about.

29

Pain Assessment: "OPQRSTU"

Assessment of pain is a crucial part in the role of nurses, and as such utilizing a problem-solving process becomes part of the equation. Pain is an unpleasant sensory and emotional experience associated with actual or potential tissue damage or described in terms of damage. Pain is subjective thus a careful assessment and evaluation is needed.

O	Onset
P	Provoking or Palliating Factors
Q	Quality
R	Region & Radiation
S	Severity
T	Time & Treatment
U	Understanding & Impact
V	Values

O: Onset
When did it begin? How long does it last (duration)? How often does it occur (time)? What were you doing when the pain started?

P: Provoking or Palliating Factors
What brings it on? What makes it better? What makes it worse?

Q: Quality
What does it feel like? Can you describe it (throbbing, stabbing, dull, etc.)?

R: Region & Radiation
Does your pain radiate? Where does it spread? Point to where it hurts the most. Where does your pain go from there?

S: Severity
What is the intensity (pain scale of 1-10, visual scales) of the symptom? Right now? At worst? Are there any other symptoms that accompany the pain?

T: Time & Treatment
When did the symptoms first begin? What medications are you currently taking for this? How effective are these? Side effects?

U: Understanding & Impact
What do you believe is causing this? How is this affecting your ADLs, you and/or your family?

V: Values
What is your goal for this symptom? What is your comfort goal or acceptable level for this symptom? Do you have any other concerns?

Isolation / Precautions Mnemonics

Droplet Precautions

Diseases included with droplet precautions:

- Pharyngeal Diphtheria
- Epiglottitis, (caused by Haemophilus influenza type b)
- Flu **(contact and droplet)**
- Meningococcal Disease: Sepsis, Pneumonia, meningitis
- Mumps (infectious parotitis)
- Pneumonia
- Mycoplasma Pneumonia
- Parvovirus B19 (erythema infectiosum or 5th disease)
- Pneumonic Plague
- Adenovirus **(contact and droplet)**
- Streptococcal pharyngitis
- Whooping Cough (pertussis)
- Rhinovirus
- Scarlet fever
- Rubella (German Measles)

Who's Adjustable Droplet Mask Stops Scary Pneumatic Fluid Parasites Plaguing Distinguished German Men? My Epic Mum's, Rhonda.

Who's: <u>Who</u>oping Cough

Adjustable: <u>Ad</u>enovirus (remember ADD contact precautions as well)

Droplet: type of precaution

Mask: PPE you must wear at all times

Stops: <u>St</u>reptococcal pharyngitis

Scary: <u>Scar</u>let fever

Pneumatic: <u>**Pneum**</u>onia

Fluid: <u>**Flu**</u> (influenza)

Parasites: **Par**vovirus B19

Plaguing: Pneumonic **Plagu**e

Distinguished: **Di**phtheria

German: **German** Measles (Rubella)

Men: **Men**ingococcal Disease: **M**eningitis, s**E**psis, p**N**emonia

My: **My**coplasma Pneumonia

Epic: **Epi**glottitis

Mum's: **Mum**ps

Rhonda: **Rh**inovirus

Airborne Precautions

Diseases included with airborne precautions:

- Chicken Pox (varicella) **(Airborne and Contact)**
- Herpes Zoster (Varicella Zoster(disseminated) Shingles **(Airborne and Contact)**
- Measles (Rubeola)
- M. Tuberculosis

Airborne Chicken Number 95 Dissected Her Tubby Mealworm

Airborne: type of isolation precaution

Chicken: <u>Chicken</u> Pox (Varicella)

Number 95: <u>N95</u> mask…special PPE you must wear at all times

Dissected **Her:** <u>Diss</u>eminated <u>Her</u>pes Zoster (Shingles)

Tubby: <u>Tub</u>erculosis

Mealworm: <u>Mea</u>sles

Contact Precautions

Diseases included with contact precautions:

- Medication-Resistant Organisms: **MRSA, VRE,** extended spectrum beta lactamase producers (**ESBLs**), Klebsiella pnemoniae carbapenemase (**KPC**)
- Diarrhea infections or of unknown origin: **C.diff, noravirus, rotavirus**.....USE SOAP AND WATER FOR HAND WASHING NOT hand-sanitizer.
  - o NOTE: Hepatitis A. (if patient is diapered or incontinent pt)..remember it is spread through stool
  - o
- Skin infection: **impetigo, lice, scabies, herpes simplex, chickenpox (airborne and contact), skin diphtheria, shingles (airborne and contact)**
- Wound infections with excessive drainage or staphylococci
- Pulmonary infections: **RSV, parainfluenza**
- Eye infection: **conjunctivitis**

Don Medical Glove/Gown With Every Contact Precaution Session

Don: Diarrhea Infections

Medical: Mediation Resistant Organisms

Gloves/Gown: PPE you must always wear at all times

With: Wound Infections

Every: Eye infections

Contact: type of isolation precaution

Precaution: Pulmonary infections

Session: Skin infections

Cardiovascular Nursing Mnemonics

Aortic regurgitation: causes

CREAM

C	Congenital
R	Rheumatic damage
E	Endocarditis
A	Aortic dissection/ Aortic root dilatation
M	Marfan's

Aortic stenosis characteristics

SAD

S	Syncope
A	Angina
D	Dyspnea

Aortic to right Subclavian path

ABC'S

A	Aortic arch gives rise to:
B	Brachiocephalic trunk
C	Left Common Carotid
S	Left Subclavian

Heart valves (right to left)

Toilet Paper My Ass, They Pay Me Alcohol, or "T"hugs "P"ush "Me" "A"round.

T	Tricuspid valve
P	Pulmonary semilunar valve
M	Mitral (bicuspid) valve
A	Aortic semilunar valve

Apex beat: abnormalities found on palpation, causes of impalpable

HILT:

H	Heaving
I	Impalpable
L	Laterally displaced
T	Thrusting/ Tapping

If it's impalpable, causes are COPD:

C	COPD
O	Obesity
P	Pleural, Pericardial effusion
D	Dextrocardia

Atrial Arrhythmias Treatment

ABCDE

A	Anticoagulants
B	Beta blockers
C	Calcium Channel Blockers
D	Digoxin
E	Electro cardioversion

Anticoagulants: To prevent embolization.

Beta blockers: To block the effects of certain hormones on the heart to slow the heart rate.

Calcium Channel Blockers: Help slow the heart rate by blocking the number of electrical impulses that pass through the AV node into the lower heart chambers (ventricles).

Digoxin: Helps slow the heart rate by blocking the number of electrical impulses that pass through the AV node into the lower heart chambers (ventricles).

Electro cardioversion: A procedure in which electric currents are used to reset the heart's rhythm back to regular pattern.

Atrial Fibrillation causes

PIRATES

P	Pulmonary: PE, COPD
I	Iatrogenic
R	Rheumatic heart: mirtral regurgitation
A	Atherosclerotic: MI, CAD
T	Thyroid: hyperthyroid
E	Endocarditis
S	Sick sinus syndrome

Atrial fibrillation management

ABCD

A	Anti-coagulate
B	Beta-block to control rate
C	Cardiovert
D	Digoxin

Beck's triad (cardiac tamponade)

3 D's

D	Distant heart sounds
D	Distended jugular veins
D	Decreased arterial pressure

Betablockers: cardioselective betablockers

Betablockers Acting Exclusively At Myocardium

B	Betaxolol
A	Acebutelol
E	Esmolol
A	Atenolol
M	Metoprolol

CHF Treatment

LMNOP

L	Lasix
M	Morphine
N	Nitrites
O	Oxygen
P	VassoPressors

CHF: causes of exacerbation

FAILURE

F	Forgot medication
A	Arrhythmia/ Anaemia
I	Ischemia/ Infarction/ Infection
L	Lifestyle: taken too much salt
U	Upregulation of CO: pregnancy, hyperthyroidism
R	Renal failure
E	Embolism: pulmonary

Complications of Myocardial Infarction

Darth Vader

D	Death
A	Arrythmia
R	Rupture(free ventricular wall/ ventricular septum/ papillary muscles)
T	Tamponade
H	Heart failure (acute or chronic)
V	Valve disease
A	Aneurysm of Ventricles
D	Dressler's Syndrome
E	thromboEmbolism (mural thrombus)
R	Recurrence/ mitral Regurgitation

Coronary artery bypass graft: indications

DUST

D	Depressed ventricular function
U	Unstable angina
S	Stenosis of the left main stem
T	Triple vessel disease

ECG: left vs. right bundle block

WiLLiaM MaRRoW

W pattern in V1-V2 and **M** pattern in V3-V6 is **L**eft bundle block.

M pattern in V1-V2 and **W** in V3-V6 is **R**ight bundle block.

Exercise ramp ECG: contraindications

RAMP

R	Recent MI
A	Aortic stenosis
M	MI in the last 7 days
P	Pulmonary hypertension

Endocarditis

FROM JANE

F	Fever
R	Roth's spots
O	Osler's nodes
M	Murmur of heart
J	Janeway lesions
A	Anemia
N	Nail hemorrhage
E	Emboli

Heart valve sequence

Try Puling My Aorta

T	Tricuspid
P	Pulmonary
M	Mitral (bicuspid)
A	Aorta

Heart blocks

If the **R** is far from **P**, then you have a **First Degree**.

Longer, longer, longer, drop! Then you have a **Wenkebach**.

if some **P**'s don't get through, then you have **Mobitz II**.

If **P**'s and **Q**'s don't agree, then you have a **Third Degree**.

Infarctions TREATMENT

INFARCTIONS

I	IV access
N	Narcotic analgesics (e.g. morphine, pethidine)
F	Facilities for defibrillation (DF)
A	Aspirin/ Anticoagulant (heparin)
R	Rest
C	Converting enzyme inhibitor
T	Thrombolysis
I	IV beta blocker
O	Oxygen 60%
N	Nitrates
S	Stool Softeners

JVP: wave form

ASK ME

A	Atrial contraction
S	Systole (ventricular contraction)
K	Klosure (closure) of tricusps, so atrial filling
M	Maximal atrial filling
E	Emptying of atrium

MI: basic management

BOOMAR

B	Bed rest
O	Oxygen
O	Opiate
M	Monitor
A	Anticoagulant
R	Reduce clot size

MI: signs and symptoms

PULSE

P	Persistent chest pains
U	Upset stomach
L	Lightheadedness
S	Shortness of breath
E	Excessive sweating

MI: therapeutic treatment

O BATMAN

O	Oxygen
B	Beta blocker
A	ASA
T	Thrombolytics (e.g. heparin)
M	Morphine
A	Ace prn
N	Nitroglycerin

MI: treatment of acute MI

COAG

C	Cyclomorph
O	Oxygen
A	Aspirin
G	Glycerol trinitrate

Murmur attributes

"IL PQRST" (person has ill PQRST heart waves)

I	Intensity
L	Loccasion
P	Pitch
Q	Quality
R	Radiation
S	Shape
T	Timing

Murmurs: innocent murmur features

8 S's

S	Soft
S	Systolic
S	Short
S	Sounds (S1 & S2) normal
S	Symptomless
S	Special tests normal (X-ray, EKG)
S	Standing/ Sitting (vary with position)
S	Sternal depression

Murmurs: louder with inspiration vs expiration

LEft sided murmurs louder with Expiration

RIght sided murmurs louder with Inspiration.

Murmurs: questions to ask

SCRIPT

S	Site
C	Character (e.g. harsh, soft, blowing)
R	Radiation
I	Intensity
P	Pitch
T	Timing

Murmurs: systolic vs. diastolic

PASS:Pulmonic & Aortic

Stenosis=Systolic.

PAID: Pulmonic & Aortic

Insufficiency=Diastolic.

Pericarditis: causes

CARDIAC RIND

C	Collagen vascular disease
A	Aortic aneurysm
R	Radiation
D	Drugs (such as hydralazine)
I	Infections
A	Acute renal failure
C	Cardiac infarction
R	Rheumatic fever
I	Injury
N	Neoplasms
D	Dressler's syndrome

Pericarditis: EKG

PericarditiS

PR depression in **p**recordial leads.

ST elevation.

Peripheral vascular insufficiency: inspection criteria

SICVD

S	Symmetry of leg musculature
I	Integrity of skin
C	Color of toenails
V	Varicose veins
D	Distribution of hair

Pulseless electrical activity: causes

PATCH MED

P	Pulmonary embolus
A	Acidosis
T	Tension pneumothorax
C	Cardiac tamponade
H	Hypokalemia/ Hyperkalemia/ Hypoxia/ Hypothermia/ Hypovolemia
M	Myocardial infarction
E	Electrolyte derangements
D	Drugs

ST elevation causes in ECG

ELEVATION

E	Electrolytes
L	LBBB
E	Early repolarization
V	Ventricular hypertrophy
A	Aneurysm
T	Treatment (e.g. pericardiocentesis)
I	Injury (AMI, contusion)
O	Osborne waves (hypothermia)
N	Non-occlusive vasospasm

Supraventricular tachycardia: treatment

ABCDE

A	Adenosine
B	Beta-blocker
C	Calcium channel antagonist
D	Digoxin
E	Excitation (vagal stimulation)

Ventricular tachycardia: treatment

LAMB

L	Lidocaine
A	Amiodarone
M	Mexiltene/ Magnesium
B	Beta-blocker

White Blood Cell Count

Never let mon

keys eat bananas

N	Neutrophils
L	Lymphocytes
M	Monocytes
E	Eosinophils
B	Basophils

Heart Blocks: "The Heart Block Poem"

Heart blocks are abnormal heart rhythm where the heart beats too slowly. In this condition, the electrical signals that tell that heart to contract are partially or totally blocked between the upper chambers (atria) and lower chambers (ventricles).

If the R is far from P then you have a **FIRST DGREE.**

Longer, Longer, Longer, Drop!! Then you have **WENCKEBACH.**

If some Ps don't get through, then you have **MOBITZ II.**

If Ps and Qs don't agree, then you have a **THIRD DGREE.**

Right-Sided Heart Failure Manifestations: "AW HEAD"

A	Anorexia and nausea
Results from the venous engorgement and venous stasis within the abdominal organs	
W	Weight gain
Due to retention of fluid.	
H	Hepatomegaly
Results from the venous engorgement of the <u>liver</u>; increased pressure may interfere with the liver's ability to function.	
E	Edema (Bipedal)
Edema usually affects the feet and ankles and worsens when the patient stands or sits for a long period.	
A	Ascites
Is the accumulation of fluid in the peritoneal cavity; increased pressure within the portal vessels forces fluid into the abdominal cavity.	
D	Distended neck vein
Increased venous pressure leads to distended neck veins.	

When the right ventricle fails in right-sided heart failure, congestion in the peripheral tissues and the viscera predominates. This occurs because the right side of the heart cannot eject blood and cannot accommodate all the blood that normally returns to it from the venous circulation. Right-sided heart failure primarily produces systemic signs and symptoms.

Left-Sided Heart Failure: "DO CHAP"

D	Dyspnea
May be precipitated by minimal to moderate activity; also occurs during rest	
O	Orthopnea
Dyspnea that develops in the recumbent position and is relieved with elevation of the head with pillows.	
C	Cough
Cough is initially dry and nonproductive. Large volume of frothy sputum, which is sometimes pink, may be produced, usually indicating severe pulmonary congestion.	
H	Hemoptysis
Pink or blood-tinged sputum may be produced.	
A	Adventitious breath sounds
May be heard in various areas of the lungs; as failure worsen, pulmonary congestion increases and crackles may be auscultated throughout the lung fields.	
P	Pulmonary congestion (crackles/rales)
Sustained high pressure in the pulmonary veins eventually forces some fluid from the blood into the surrounding microscopic air sacs (alveoli), which transfer oxygen to the bloodstream.	

Pulmonary congestion usually occurs in left-sided heart failure; when the left ventricle cannot effectively pump blood out of the ventricle into the aorta and to the systemic circulation. Blood volume and pressure in the left atrium increases which decreases blood flow from the pulmonary vessels. Pulmonary venous blood volume and pressure increase, forcing fluid from the pulmonary capillaries into the pulmonary tissues and alveoli, causing pulmonary interstitial edema and impaired gas exchange.

Management of Heart Failure: "DAD BOND CLASH"

Management of HF are to relieve patient symptoms, to improve functional status and quality of life, and to extend survival. Medical management depends on the type, severity, and cause of HF — it can include reducing the workload of the heart by reducing preload and afterload; elimination of contributing factors such as hypertension. Remember the mnemonic "DAD BOND CLASH" for the medical management of heart failure.

D	Digitalis
A	ACE Inhibitors
D	Dobutamine
B	Beta-blockers
O	Oxygen
N	Nitrates
D	Diuretics
C	Calcium Channel Blockers
L	Lifestyle Changes
A	Angiotensin II Receptor Blockers
S	Sodium restriction
H	Hydralazine

D: Digitalis
Increases the force of myocardial contraction and slows conduction through the atrioventricular node; improves contractility, increasing left ventricular output, and enhances diuresis.

A: ACE Inhibitors
Promotes vasodilation and diuresis by decreasing afterload and preload, ultimately decreasing the workload of the heart.

D: Dobutamine
IV medication administered to patients with significant left ventricular dysfunction and hypo perfusion; stimulates the beta-1-adrenergic receptors.

B: Beta-blockers
Reduces mortality and morbidity in HF by reducing the adverse effects from constant stimulation of the sympathetic nervous system.

O: Oxygen
Oxygen may be necessary as HF progresses; need is based on the degree of pulmonary congestion and resulting hypoxia.

N: Nitrates
Causes venous dilation, which reduces the amount of blood return to the heart and lowers preload.

D: Diuretics
To remove excess extracellular fluid by increasing the rate of urine produced in patients with fluid overload.

C: Calcium Channel Blockers
Causes vasodilation, reducing systemic vascular resistance.

L: Lifestyle Changes
Restriction of dietary sodium, avoidance of excess fluid intake, weight reduction, and regular exercise.

A: Angiotensin II Receptor Blockers
ARBs block the effects of angiotensin II at its receptor; have similar hemodynamic effects as of ACE inhibitors. Serves as alternative for patients who cannot tolerate ACE inhibitors.

S: Sodium restriction
A low-sodium diet (2 to 3 g/day) diet and avoidance of drinking excess amounts of fluid is recommended.
H: Hydralazine
Lowers systemic vascular resistance and left ventricular afterload.

Hypertension Complications "5 C's of Hypertension Complications"

The excessive pressure on the artery walls caused by hypertension or high blood pressure can damage the blood vessels, as well as organs in the body. The higher the blood pressure and the longer it goes uncontrolled, the greater the damage. With time, hypertension increases the risk of heart disease, kidney disease, and stroke.

C	Coronary Artery Disease
C	Chronic Renal Failure
C	Congestive Heart Failure
C	Cardiac Arrest
C	Cerebrovascular Accident

C: Coronary Artery Disease
Can lead to narrowing of blood vessels making them more likely to block from blood clots or fat breaking off from the lining of the blood vessel wall; also weakens the walls.

C: Chronic Renal Failure
Constant high blood pressure can damage small blood vessels in the kidneys making it not to function properly.

C: Congestive Heart Failure
Pumping blood against the higher pressure in the vessels causes the heart muscles to thicken. Eventually, the heart muscles may have a hard time pumping enough blood to meet the physiologic needs of the body leading to heart failure.

C: Cardiac Arrest
High blood pressure can cause CAD, damaged arteries cannot deliver enough oxygen to other parts of the body eventually leading to heart attack.

C: Cerebrovascular Accident
Hypertension leads to atherosclerosis and hardening of the large arteries. This, in turn, can lead to blockage of small blood vessels in the brain. It can also weaken the blood vessels in the brain causing them to balloon and burst.

Immediate Treatment of a Myocardial Infarction Client "MONA TASS"

MONA is a mnemonic that stands for: Morphine, Oxygen, Nitrates, and Aspirin. These are the four primary interventions that are performed when treating a patient with Heart Attack/Myocardial Infarction (MI). However, MONA does not represent the order in which you should administer these treatments as a nurse. It is a mnemonic intended to help you remember the components of MI treatment, not the prioritization of them.

M	Morphine
O	Oxygen
N	Nitroglycerine
A	Aspirin
T	Thrombolytics
A	Anticoagulants
S	Stool Softeners
S	Sedatives

M: Morphine
Analgesic drugs such as morphine are to reduce pain and anxiety, also has other beneficial effects as a vasodilator and decreases the workload of the heart by reducing preload and afterload.

O: Oxygen
To provide and improve oxygenation of ischemic myocardial tissue; enforced together with bedrest to help reduce myocardial oxygen consumption. Given via nasal cannula at 2 to 4 L/min.

N: Nitroglycerine

First-line of treatment for angina pectoris and acute MI; causes vasodilation and increases blood flow to the myocardium.

A: Aspirin

Aspirin prevents the formation of thromboxane A2 which causes platelets to aggregate and arteries to constrict. The earlier the patient receives ASA after symptom onset, the greater the potential benefit.

T: Thrombolytics

To dissolve the thrombus in a coronary artery, allowing blood to flow through again, minimizing the size of the infarction and preserving ventricular function; given in some patients with MI.

A: Anticoagulants

Given to prevent clots from becoming larger and block coronary arteries. They are usually given with other anticlotting medicines to help prevent or reduce heart muscle damage.

S: Stool Softeners

Given to avoid intense straining that may trigger arrhythmias or another cardiac arrest.

S: Sedatives

In order to limit the size of infarction and give rest to the patient. Valium or an equivalent is usually given.

Myocardial Infarction Management: "INFARCTIONS"

Goals of treatment during MI are to minimize myocardial damage, preserve myocardial function, and prevent complications. These goals can be achieved by reperfusion the area with the emergency use of thrombolytic medications or by PCI. Reducing myocardial oxygen demand, and increasing oxygen supply with medications, oxygen administration and bed rest can minimize myocardial damage.

I	IV access
N	Narcotic analgesics
F	Facilities for defibrillation (DF)
A	Aspirin
R	Rest
C	Converting enzyme inhibitor
T	Thrombolytic
I	IV beta blocker
O	Oxygen
N	Nitrates
S	Stool Softeners

I: IV access
Two IV lines are placed usually to ensure that access is available for administering emergency medications.

N: Narcotic analgesics
Morphine is the analgesic of choice for MI and is administered in IV boluses to reduce pain and anxiety; reduces preload and afterload and relaxes bronchioles to enhance oxygenation.

F: Facilities for defibrillation (DF)
Have the crash cart available and ready.

A: Aspirin
Inhibits platelet aggregation. Treatment should be initiated immediately and continued for years.

R: Rest
Bed rest promotes comfort and healing.

C: Converting enzyme inhibitor
ACE-inhibitors lowers the blood pressure and the kidneys excrete sodium and fluid.

T: Thrombolytic
Administered via IV to dissolve the thrombus in a coronary artery, allowing blood reperfusion, minimizing the size of the infarction and preserving ventricular function.

I: IV beta blocker
Long-term therapy with beta-blockers decreases the future incidences of cardiac events.

O: Oxygen
Administer at a modest flow rate for 2 to 3 LPM.

N: Nitrates
To increase cardiac output and reduce myocardial workload; relieves pain by redistributing blood to ischemic areas of the myocardium.

S: Stool Softeners
To prevent straining during defecation, which causes vagal stimulation and may slow the heart rate.

Myocardial Infarction Nursing Management

"BEE CAB SCORE"

Nursing care for patients who suffered MI is directed towards detecting complications, preventing further myocardial damage, and promoting comfort, rest, and emotional well-being.

B	Bed rest
E	ECG Monitoring
E	Emotional support
C	Cluster/Organize Patient Care
A	Anti-embolism stockings
B	Bedside commode
S	Stool Softener
C	Cardiac Rehabilitation Program
O	Oxygen therapy
R	Range-of-motion Exercises
E	Educate and inform

B: Bed rest
Bed rest helps reduce myocardial oxygen consumption.

E: ECG Monitoring
Frequently monitor ECG to detect rate changes or arrhythmias; place rhythm strips in the patient's chart for evaluation.

E: Emotional support
Provide support and help reduce stress and anxiety; administer tranquilizers as needed.

C: Cluster/Organize Patient Care
To maximize periods of uninterrupted rest.

A: Anti-embolism stockings
Can help prevent veno-stasis and thrombophlebitis.

B: Bedside commode
Allow use of bedside commode and provide privacy as much as possible.

S: Stool Softener
To prevent straining during defecation causing vagal stimulation and slow heart rate.

C: Cardiac Rehabilitation Program
Includes education regarding heart disease, exercise, and emotional support for the patient and the family.

O: Oxygen therapy
Increases available oxygen; set at 2-3 LPM.

R: Range-of-motion Exercises
Provides physical activity for the patient; if immobilized, turn him often.

E: Educate and inform
Explain procedures and answer questions.

Cardiopulmonary Bypass Complications

"4 H's of CBP"

Cardiopulmonary bypass (CPB) mechanically circulates and oxygenates blood for the body while bypassing the heart and lungs. CPB maintains perfusion to body organs and tissues and allows the surgeon to complete the anastomosis in a motionless, bloodless, surgical field. CPB is not benign and there are a number of associated problems; use is limited to several hours.

H	
H	Hypothermia
H	Hemodilution
H	Heparinization
H	Head or "Pumohead"

H: Hypothermia
Because blood is cooled during CPB to slow the body's basal metabolic rate.

H: Hemodilution
Due to administration of isotonic crystalloid solution during the procedure.

H: Heparinization
Heparin is used to prevent clotting and thrombus formation in the bypass circuit when blood comes in contact with the surface of the tubing.

H: Head or "Pumphead"
AKA postperfusion syndrome, include defects associated with attention, concentration, short term memory, fine motor function, and speed of mental and motor responses.

The "3 D's" Cardiac Tamponade (Beck's Triad)

In cardiac tamponade, blood or fluid collects in the pericardium, the sac surrounding the heart. Pericardial fluid may accumulate slowly without causing any noticeable symptoms until a large amount accumulates. However, a rapidly developing effusion can stretch the pericardium to its maximum size and, because of increased pericardial pressure, reduce venous return to the heart and decrease CO. It often has three characteristic signs that the physician will recognize during a physical exam. These signs are commonly referred to as "Beck's Triad" or The 3 D's.

D	Distant or muffled heart sounds
D	Distended jugular veins
D	Decreased pulse pressure

For Endocarditis, you can remember FAME.

F	Fever
A	Anemia
M	Murmur
E	Endocarditis

74

To be able to remember the cause of heart Murmur, think of SPAMS.

S	Stenosis of a valve
P	Partial obstruction
A	Aneurysm
M	Mitral
S	Septal defect

Remember FAST for the signs of a stroke.

F	Face
A	Arms
S	Speech
T	Time

Pharmacology Nursing Mnemonics

Lidocaine Toxicity: "SAMS"

Lidocaine is a class IB antiarrhythmic used as a second-line agent and after myocardial infarction. The therapeutic drug range for lidocaine is 1.5-5.0 mcg/mL. While generally safe, lidocaine can be toxic if administered inappropriately, and in some cases may cause unintended reactions even when properly administered. Lidocaine toxicity is seen at levels greater than 5 mcg/mL. Remember the mnemonic SAMS for signs and symptoms of lidocaine toxicity.

S	Slurred speech
A	Altered central nervous system
M	Muscle twitching
S	Seizures

Medication Administration Checklist: "TRAMP"

Nurses are primarily involved in the administration of medication across various settings. They are primarily involved in both dispensing and preparation of medication. Research on medical administration errors (MAEs) shows an error rate of 60%, 34% mainly in the form of wrong time, wrong rate, or wrong dose. Before dispensing medication, ensure the correct **TRAMP**.

T	Time
R	Route
A	Amount
M	Medication
P	Patient

T: Time
Check the order for when it would be given and when was the last time it was given.

R: Route
Check the order if it's through oral, IV, SQ, IM, or etc.

A: Amount
Check the medication sheet and the doctor's order before medicating. Be aware of the difference of an adult and a pediatric dose.

M: Medication
Check and verify if it's the right name and form. Beware of look-alike and sound-alike medication names.

P: Patient
Ask the name of the client and check his/her ID band before giving the medication. Even if you know that patient's name, you still need to ask just to verify.

Serious Complications of Oral Birth Control Pills

"SEA CASH"

Some women experience side effects with "the pill" such as irregular periods, nausea, headaches, or weight change. If she experiences the side effects with the acronym SEA CASH, calling the help of a medical provider or visiting an emergency room immediately is recommended as they may signify a serious condition.

S	Severe leg pain
E	Eye problems
A	Abdominal pain
C	Chest pain
A	Acne
S	Swelling of ankles and feet
H	Headaches which are severe

Emergency Drugs to "LEAN" on

In the hospital setting, emergencies typically occur in emergency departments (EDs) and intensive care units (ICUs). The goal of using these common emergency drugs is to prevent the patient from deteriorating to an arrest situation.

L	Lidocaine
E	Epinephrine
A	Atropine Sulfate
N	Narcan

L:Lidocaine
ACTION: Suppresses automaticity of ventricular cells, decreasing diastolic depolarization and increasing ventricular fibrillation threshold. Produces local anesthesia by reducing sodium permeability of sensory nerves, which blocks impulse generation and conduction. USES: Ventricular arrhythmias, topical/local anesthetic

E:Epinephrine
ACTION: Stimulates alpha- and beta-adrenergic receptors, causing relaxation of cardiac and bronchial smooth muscle and dilation of skeletal muscles. USES: Bronchodilation; anaphylaxis; hypersensitivity reaction; Acute asthma attack; Chronic simple glaucoma

A:AtropineSulfate
ACTION: Inhibits acetylcholine at parasympathetic neuroeffector junction of smooth muscle and cardiac muscle, blocking sinoatrial (SA) and atrioventricular (AV) nodes to increase impulse conduction and raise heart rate. USES: Decreases respiratory secretions, treats sinus bradycardia, reverses effects of anticholinesterase medication

N:Narcan
ACTION: Naloxone is used to treat an opioid emergency such as an overdose or a possible overdose of a narcotic medicine. USES: Opioid-induced toxicity; opioid-induced respiratory depression; used in neonates to counteract or treat effects from narcotics given to mother during labor

Drugs for Bradycardia & Hypotension: "IDEA"

Beta blockers reduce circulating catecholamine levels, decreasing both the heart rate and blood pressure. Typically, atropine is the drug of choice for symptomatic bradycardia. Antiarrhythmic and digoxin may also be used.

I	Isoproterenol
D	Dopamine
E	Epinephrine
A	Atropine Sulfate

I:Isoproterenol
Acts on beta2-adrenergic receptors, causing relaxation of bronchial smooth muscle; acts on beta1-adrenergic receptors in heart, causing positive inotropic and chronotropic effects and increasing cardiac output. Also lowers peripheral vascular resistance in skeletal muscle and inhibits antigen-induced histamine release.

D:Dopamine
Causes norepinephrine release (mainly on dopaminergic receptors), leading to vasodilation of renal and mesenteric arteries. Also exerts inotropic effects on heart, which increases the heart rate, blood flow, myocardial contractility, and stroke volume.

E:Epinephrine
Stimulates alpha- and beta-adrenergic receptors, causing relaxation of cardiac and bronchial smooth muscle and dilation of skeletal muscles. Also decreases aqueous humor production, increases aqueous outflow, and dilates pupils by contracting dilator muscle.

A:AtropineSulfate
Acts on beta2-adrenergic receptors, causing relaxation of bronchial smooth muscle; acts on beta1-adrenergic receptors in heart, causing positive inotropic and chronotropic effects and increasing cardiac output. Also lowers peripheral vascular resistance in skeletal muscle and inhibits antigen-induced histamine release.

Thiazides Indications: "CHIC"

Thiazides affect the level of the nephron, inhibiting the reabsorption of sodium by the tubules at the cortical diluting segment of the nephron. The thiazides are the most commonly used oral diuretics and are widely used in the therapy of hypertension and congestive heart failure, as well as the treatment of edema due to local, renal and hepatic causes. Remember CHIC to thiazides indications!

C	Congestive Heart Failure
H	Hypertension
I	Insipidus
C	Calcium calculi

Parkinson's Medications: "ALBM"

There are many medications available to treat the symptoms of Parkinson's, although none yet that actually reverse the effects of the disease. Most Parkinson's disease treatments aim to restore the proper balance of the neurotransmitters acetylcholine and dopamine by increasing dopamine levels. It is common for people with PD to take a variety of these medications. To familiarize yourself with the common drugs used for PD, remember the mnemonic: "Ali Loves Boxing Matches". The former champion boxer Muhammad Ali was diagnosed with Parkinson's in 1984 at the age of 42, and is one of the most high-profile people battling the condition.

L	Levodopa
A	Amantadine
M	MAO Inhibitors
B	Bromocriptine

L: Levodopa

Levodopa is the drug most often prescribed. The body metabolizes it to produce dopamine. Giving dopamine directly is ineffective, because the brain 's natural defense blocks it from being used by the body. To suppress nausea and other possible side effects, levodopa is used in conjunction with a related drug called carbidopa.

A: Amantadine

It improves muscle control and reduces stiffness in Parkinson's disease; allows more normal movements of the body as the disease symptoms are reduced. Amantadine is also used to treat stiffness and shaking caused by certain medicines that are used to treat nervous, mental, and emotional conditions.

M: MAO Inhibitors

MAO-B inhibitors also block the action of an enzyme that breaks down dopamine. They may be taken alone early in Parkinson's disease or with other drugs as the disease progresses. MAO Inhibitors are often used alone because combining them with other drugs can cause unwanted side effects.

B: Bromocriptine

It improves the ability to move and decrease shakiness (tremor), stiffness, slowed movement, and unsteadiness. It may also decrease the number of episodes of not being able to move ("on-off syndrome").

Morphine Side Effects: "MORPHINE"

Morphine interacts with opioid receptor sites, primarily in limbic system, thalamus, and spinal cord. This interaction alters neurotransmitter release, altering perception of and tolerance for pain. If side-effects occur, opioid rotation may be used for managing opioid-induced adverse effects.

M	Myosis
O	Out of it (sedation)
R	Respiratory depression
P	Pneumonia (aspiration)
H	Hypotension
I	Infrequency (constipation, urinary retention)
N	Nausea
E	Emesis

Atrial Arrhythmias: "ABCDE"

Atrial fibrillation is the most common sustained atrial arrhythmia. A variety of medicines are available to restore normal heart rhythm. A beta-blocker, such as bisoprolol or atenolol, or a calcium channel blocker, such as verapamil or diltiazem, will be prescribed. Digoxin may be added to help control the heart rate further. In some cases, amiodarone may be tried, or simply remember the mnemonic ABCDE.

A	Anticoagulants
B	Beta blockers
C	Calcium Channel Blockers
D	Digoxin
E	Electro cardioversion

A: Anticoagulants
To prevent embolization.

B: Beta blockers
To block the effects of certain hormones on the heart to slow the heart rate.

C: Calcium Channel Blockers
Help slow the heart rate by blocking the number of electrical impulses that pass through the AV node into the lower heart chambers (ventricles).

D: Digoxin
Digoxin helps slow the heart rate by blocking the number of electrical impulses that pass through the AV node into the lower heart chambers (ventricles).

E: Electro cardioversion
A procedure in which electric currents are used to reset the heart's rhythm back to regular pattern.

Ventricular Arrhythmias: "SLAP"

Treatment for ventricular arrhythmias depends on the symptoms, and the type of heart disorder. Some people may not need treatment. If ventricular tachycardia becomes an emergency situation, it may require CPR and electrical defibrillation or cardioversion (electric shock). And to prevent the arrhythmia from recurring, anti-arrhythmic medications such as procainamide, amiodarone, lidocaine, or sotalol are given through a vein.

S	Anticoagulants
L	Beta blockers
A	Calcium Channel Blockers
P	Digoxin

S: Sotalol
Blocks stimulation of cardiac beta1-adrenergic and pulmonary, vascular, beta2-adrenergic receptor sites. This action reduces cardiac output and blood pressure, depresses sinus heart rate, and prolongs refractory period in atria and ventricles.

L: Lidocaine
Suppresses automaticity of ventricular cells, decreasing diastolic depolarization and increasing ventricular fibrillation threshold.

A: Amiodarone
Prolongs duration and refractory period of action potential. Slows electrical conduction, electrical impulse generation from sinoatrial node, and conduction through accessory pathways.

P: Procainamide
Decreases myocardial excitability by inhibiting conduction velocity. Also depresses myocardial contractility.

For the treatment of Myocardial Infarction, you can think of the name MONA.

M	Morphine
O	Oxygen
N	Nitroglycerine
A	Asa

The drugs that are used in the treatment of HIV can be memorized with ZZLSD.

Z	Zidovudine
Z	Zalcitabine
L	Lamivudine
S	Stavudine
D	Didanosine

Remember MADD DOG for the treatment of congestive heart failure.

M	Morphine
A	Aminophylline
D	Digoxin
D	Dopamine
D	Diuretics
O	Oxygen
G	Gasses (gasses is for monitoring the arterial blood gasses)

Maternal and Child Health Nursing Mnemonics

Severe Pre-Eclampsia: *HELLP Syndrome*

HELLP syndrome is a life-threatening pregnancy complication usually considered to be a variant of preeclampsia. Both conditions usually occur during the later stages of pregnancy, or sometimes after childbirth.

H	Hemolysis
E	Elevated
L	Liver enzymes
L	Low
P	Platelet Count

Postpartum Assessment: *"BUBBLE-HE"*
Nurses need to be aware of the normal physiologic and psychological changes that take place in women's bodies and minds in order to provide comprehensive care during this period. The postpartum period covers the time period from birth until approximately six weeks after delivery. So it is important to remember the mnemonic BUBBLE-HE to denote the components of the postpartum maternal nursing assessment.

B	Breast
U	Uterus
B	Bowel
B	Bladder
L	Lochia
E	Episiotmy
H	Homan's sign
E	Emotional Status

Fetal Non-Stress Test: *"NNN"*

A nonstress test is a common prenatal test used to check on a baby's health. Results of a nonstress test are considered reactive or nonreactive. Results are considered normal (reactive) if the baby's heartbeat accelerates to a certain level twice or more. If the baby's heartbeat doesn't meet the criteria described, the results are considered nonreactive.

N	Non-Reactive
N	Non-Stress Test Is
N	Not Good

The APGAR score is used to gauge the health of a baby at 1 minute and 5 minutes after being born.

A	**Appearance: Is the baby blue/pale, blue/pink, or pink?**
P	Pulse: Is the pulse absent, under 100, or greater than 100?
G	Grimace: Response to stimulation
A	Activity: Flexing of the limbs
R	Respiration: Is there crying and is it weak or strong?

Fetal Wellbeing Assessment Tests: *"ALONE"*

Assessment of fetal well-being is crucial not only for high risk patients but also for other pregnant women who might develop unexpected complications in the course of otherwise normal pregnancies. The primary goal of antenatal evaluation is to identify fetuses at risk for intrauterine injury and death so that intervention and timely delivery can prevent progression to stillbirth.

A	Amniocentesis
L	L/S Ratio
O	Oxytocin Test
N	nonstress test
E	Estriol Level

Amniocentesis is a prenatal test where a small amount of amniotic fluid is removed from the sac surrounding the fetus for testing. Different tests can be performed on a sample, but it is used mainly to look for certain types of birth defects, such as Down syndrome, a chromosomal abnormality.

The lecithin–sphingomyelin ratio (aka L-S or L/S ratio) is a test of fetal amniotic fluid to assess for fetal lung immaturity.
Oxytocin Test or Challenge (a.k.a. Contraction Test) involves the intravenous administration of exogenous oxytocin to the pregnant woman. The target is to achieve around three contractions every ten minutes.

A nonstress test is used to evaluate a fetus' health before birth and provides useful information how the fetus' oxygen supply by checking its heart rate and how it responds to the fetus' movement.
Levels of estriol in the blood is used in maternal serum triple or quadruple screening test that is done between 15 and 20 weeks. The levels of the substances measured helps estimate the chance that the baby may have certain problems or birth defects.

Episiotomy Healing Evaluation: *"REEDDA"*

If the mother had an episiotomy or vaginal tear during delivery, the wound might hurt for a few weeks. Extensive tears might take longer to heal. The patient will have a vaginal discharge (lochia) for a number of weeks after delivery. Expect a bright red, heavy flow of blood for the first few days. The discharge will gradually taper off, becoming watery and changing from pink or brown to yellow or white. So it is always important to check for REEDA.

R	REDNESS
E	EDEMA
E	ECCHYMOSIS
D	DISCHARGES
D	DRAINAGE
A	APPROXIMATION

Fetal Accelerations and Decelerations: *"VEAL CHOP"*

Variable decelerations are associated with cord compression (V and C). Early decelerations are associated with head compression. This is generally a benign event (E and H). Accelerations are associated with oxygenation, which explains why they're generally a good prognostic factor (A and O). Late decelerations* are associated with placental insufficiency (L and P). The trick to this mnemonic is writing it so each letter is associated with the one beneath it, or the other way around.

Variable Deceleration	V	C	Cord Compression
Early Deceleration	E	H	Head Compression
Acceleration	A	O	OKAY
Late Deceleration	L	P	Placental Insufficiency

Chorionic Villi Sampling & Alpha-fetoprotein

"Chorionic" has 9 letters and CVS is performed at 9 weeks' gestation. "Alpha Fetoprotein" has 16 letters and is measured at 16 weeks' gestation.

Chorionic villus sampling and Alpha-fetoprotein	
9 & 16	
Chorionic	has 9 letters and CVS is performed at 9 weeks gestation
Alpha-fetoprotein	" has 16 letters and is measured at 16 weeks gestation.

Chorionic villus sampling (CVS) is a first-trimester (10 to 12 weeks) alternative to amniocentesis for prenatal diagnosis of genetic abnormalities. This procedure is accomplished by needle aspiration of a sample of chorionic villi, either by the trans cervical or transabdominal route.

Alpha-fetoprotein is a fetal protein produced in the yolk sac during the first 6 weeks of gestation and later by the fetal liver. AFP is found in the amniotic fluid and maternal serum. If the fetus has neural tube defect, AFP levels are elevated.

Prenatal Care Assessment: *"ABCDEF"*

The first prenatal visit is a time to establish rapport and baseline data relevant to the patient's health. This begins with obtaining a health history, including screening for any presence of teratogens and concerns the woman may be experiencing. If you are lost with your assessment, remember the nursing mnemonic "ABCDEF" for the possible areas you can ask.

A	Amniotic fluid leakage
B	Bleeding vaginally
C	Contractions
D	Dysuria
E	Edema
F	Fetal movement (quickening)

A: Amniotic fluid leakage
Check whether amniotic fluid is clear, blood-tinged (pink), green, or brown. A woman can tell the difference between urine and amniotic fluid because the fluid keeps leaking and she can't control its release.

B: Bleeding vaginally
Bleeding during pregnancy can happen any time from conception to the end of pregnancy. Any bleeding or spotting can be a sign of pregnancy where the fertilized egg develops outside the uterus (ectopic). An untreated ectopic pregnancy can be life-threatening for the woman.

C: Contractions
A pregnant mother may experience them from as early as six weeks into pregnancy to the very end, or not at all. These contractions typically feel like a tightening or hardening across the abdomen and should be irregular and totally painless.

D: Dysuria
Pregnant women are also more susceptible to urinary tract infections. Be careful not to confuse increased frequency of urination with a bladder infection (cystitis). If a pregnant woman notices that she is urinating more frequently, that urination is painful (dysuria), or that she has a fever, she may have an infection.

E: Edema
Edema is when excess fluid collects in the tissue. It's normal to have a certain amount of swelling during pregnancy because of water retention. Edema is most likely to trouble during the third trimester. It may be particularly severe for women with excessive amniotic fluid or those carrying multiples.

F: Fetal movement (quickening)
This can usually be felt between 16 and 23 weeks; movements are intermittent and infrequent.

Abdominal Pain Causes During Pregnancy:

"LARA CROFT"

Intermittent abdominal discomfort or pain is a common pregnancy complaint. While itself may present to be harmless, it can also be a sign of a serious problem. There can be many causes for abdominal pain especially during pregnancy, remember the nursing mnemonic "LARA CROFT" to remind you.

L	Labor
A	Abruptio Placenta
R	Rupture (e.g., ectopic/uterine rupture)
A	Abortion (Spontaneous)
C	Cholestasis
R	Rectus sheath hematoma (RSH)
O	Ovarian tumor
F	Fibroids
T	Torsion of the uterus

L: Labor
Labor contractions usually cause discomfort or a dull ache in a pregnant woman's back and lower abdomen, along with pressure in the pelvis.

A: Abruptio Placenta
The premature separation of placenta from the uterus and typically presents with bleeding, uterine contractions, and fetal distress. Puts mother and fetus in serious danger if left untreated.

R: Rupture (e.g., ectopic/uterine rupture)
Ruptured ectopic pregnancy often results in internal bleeding and intense abdominal pain.
Rupture of the uterus results in bleeding, rupture of the amniotic sac; it is a serious emergency.

A: Abortion (Spontaneous)
Spontaneous abortion (a.k.a. miscarriage) is the unintentional expulsion of an embryo or fetus before the 24th week of gestation; manifests with abdominal cramps and vaginal bleeding.

C: Cholestasis
Cholestasis is the impairment of bile flow from the liver that can trigger intense itching and abdominal pain. It poses no risk for the mother but can be dangerous for the developing baby.

R: Rectus sheath hematoma (RSH)
It is a rare hematoma within the rectus sheath that produces a painful, tender swelling that can mimic an intraperitoneal mass with features of an acute abdomen.

O: Ovarian tumor
Ovarian cysts typically occur in the second trimester and typically do not pose risks to the mother or fetus; can naturally resolve themselves before or soon after childbirth.

F: Fibroids
Fibroids are benign tumors that originate in the uterus and are composed of the same smooth muscle fibers as the myometrium; usually poses no problems during pregnancy.

T: Torsion of the uterus
It is the rotation of more than 45 degrees around the long axis of the uterus; manifests with severe abdominal pain, tense uterus, and fetal distress. It may be due to structural abnormalities in the pelvis.

Preeclampsia Classic Triad:

*"PRE"*eclampsia

Preeclampsia is a complication characterized by high blood pressure and signs of damage to another organ system (usually the kidneys). The condition usually begins after 20 weeks of pregnancy in a woman whose blood pressure had been normal. Even a slight rise in blood pressure may be a sign of preeclampsia.

P	Proteinuria
R	Rising blood pressure
E	Edema

P: Proteinuria
Proteinuria is defined as > 300 mg/24 h. Alternatively, proteinuria is diagnosed based on a protein: creatinine ratio ≥ 0.3 or a dipstick reading of 1+. Absence of proteinuria on less accurate tests (eg, urine dipstick testing, routine urinalysis) does not rule out preeclampsia.

R: Rising blood pressure
High blood pressure may develop slowly, but more commonly it has a sudden onset. Blood pressure that is 140/90 millimeters of mercury (mm Hg) or greater — documented on two occasions, at least four hours apart — is abnormal.

E: Edema
Sudden weight gains and swelling (particularly in the face and hands) often manifests; pitting edema-an unusual swelling, particularly of the hands, feet, or face, notable by leaving an indentation when pressed on.

Anesthesia Nursing Mnemonics

Anesthesia machine/room check

MS MAID

M	Monitors (EKG, SpO2, EtCO2, etc.)
S	Suction
M	Machine check (according to ASA guidelines)
A	Airway equipment (ETT, laryngoscope, oral/nasal airway)
I	IV equipment
D	Drugs (emergency, inductions, NMBs, etc.)

Endotracheal intubation: diagnosis of poor bilateral breath sounds after intubation

DOPE

D	Displaced (usually right mainstem, pyreform fossa, etc.)
O	Obstruction (kinked or bitten tube, mucous plug, etc.)
P	Pneumothorax (collapsed lung)
E	Esophagus

General anesthesia: equipment checks prior to inducing

MALES

M	Masks
A	Airways
L	Laryngoscopes
E	Endotracheal tubes
S	Suction/ Stylette, bougie

Spinal anesthesia agents

"Little Boys Prefer Toys"

L	Lidocaine
B	Bupivicaine
P	Procaine
T	Tetracaine

Xylocaine: where not to use with epinephrine

"Ears, Nose, Hose, Fingers and Toes"

Vasoconstrictive effects of xylocaine with epinephrine are helpful in providing hemostasis while suturing. However, may cause local ischemic necrosis in distal structures such as the digits, tip of nose, penis, ears. "Digital PEN" - Digits, Penis, ear, nose.

Behavioral science Psychiatric Nursing Mnemonics

Depression: major episode characteristics

SPACE DIGS

S	Sleep disruption
P	Psychomotor retardation
A	Appetite change
C	Concentration loss
E	Energy loss
D	Depressed mood
I	Interest wanes
G	Guilt
S	Suicidal tendencies

Depression: DSM-V Criteria for Major Depressive Disorder

"SIG E CAPS"

S	Sleep disturbances
I	Interest decreased (anhedonia)
G	Guilt and/or feelings of worthlessness
E	Energy decreased
C	Concentration problems
A	Appetite/weight changes
P	Psychomotor agitation or retardation
S	Suicidal ideation

Gain: primary vs. secondary vs. tertiary

Primary	Patient's Psyche improved.
Secondary	Symptom Sympathy for patient.
Tertiary	Therapist's gain

Kubler-Ross dying process: stages

"'Death Always Brings Great Acceptance"

D	Denial
A	Anger
B	Bargaining
G	Grieving
A	Acceptance

Middle adolescence (14-17 years): characteristics

"HERO"

H	Heterosexual crushes/ Homosexual Experience
E	Education regarding short term benefits
R	Risk taking
O	Omnipotence

Narcolepsy: symptoms, epidemiology

"CHAP"

C	Cataplexy
H	Hallucinations
A	Attacks of sleep
P	Paralysis on waking

Usual presentation is a young male, hence "chap"

Suicide: risk screening

"SAD PERSONS" scale

SAD

S	Cataplexy
A	Hallucinations
D	Attacks of sleep

PERSONS

P	Previous attempt
E	Ethanol abuse
R	Rational thinking loss
S	Social support problems
O	Organised plan
N	No spouse
S	Sickness (chronic illness)

Sleep stages: features:

DElta waves during DEepest sleep (stages 3 & 4, slow-wave).
dREaM during REM sleep.

Impotence causes

"PLANE"

P	Psychogenic: performance anxiety
L	Libido: decreased with androgen deficiency, drugs
A	Autonomic neuropathy: impede blood flow redirection
N	Nitric oxide deficiency: impaired synthesis, decreased blood pressure
E	Erectile reserve: can't maintain an erection

Male erectile dysfunction (MED): biological causes

"MED"

M	Medicines (propranalol, methyldopa, SSRI, etc.)
E	Ethanol
D	Diabetes mellitus

Mania is one of the primary symptoms of bipolar disorder. It can also be the side effect from the use of prescription medications as well as some illicit drugs. **DIG FAST** is the acronym for the symptoms of mania.

D	Distractibility
I	Indiscretion or excessive Involvement in pleasurable activities
G	Grandiosity
F	Flight of ideas
A	Activity increase
S	Sleep deficit (meaning, there is a decrease in the need for sleep)
T	Talkativeness

Endocrine Nursing Mnemonics

Diabetes Complications

KNIVES

K	Kidney – nephropathy
N	Neuromuscular – peripheral neuropathy, mononeuritis, amyotrophy
I	Infective – UTIs, TB
V	Vascular – coronary/cerebrovascular/peripheral artery disease
E	Eye – cataracts, retinopathy
S	Skin – lipohypertrophy/lipoatrophy, necrobiosis lipoidica

Anatomy Mnemonics

Afferent vs efferent

Afferent connection arrives *and an* efferent connection exits.

Anterior leg muscles

"The Hospitals Are Not Dirty Places"

T	Tibialis anterior
H	extensor Hallucis longus
A	anterior tibial Artery
N	deep fibular Nerve
D	extensor Digitorum longus
P	Peronius tertius [aka fibularis tertius]

Brachial plexus
Remember To Drink Cold Beer - Roots, Trunks, Divisions, Cords, Branches
Posterior cord branches
STAR - subscapular (upper and lower), thoracodorsal, axillary, radial
RATS- Radial nerve, Axillary nerve, Thoracodorsal nerve, Subscapular (Upper & Lower) nerve.
ULTRA - upper subscapular, lower subscapular, thoracodorsal, radial, axillary

ULNAR- **U**pper subscapular nerve, **L**ower subscapular nerve, **N**erve to latissimus dorsi, **A**xillary nerve, **R**adial nerve.
Lateral Cord Branches
LLM "Lucy Loves Me" - lateral pectoral, lateral root of the median nerve, musculocutaneous
Love Me Latha (**LML**) - **L**ateral pectoral nerve, **M**usculocutaneous nerve, **L**ateral root of Median Nerve.
Look My Lancer-Lateral pectoral nerve, Musculocutaneous nerve,Lateral root of Median nerve.

Medial Cord Branches

MMMUM "Most Medical Men Use Morphine" - medial pectoral, medial cutaneous nerve of arm, medial cutaneous nerve of forearm, ulnar, medial root of the median nerve
"Money Makes Many Men Unhappy" - Medial pectoral nerve, Medial cutaneous nerve of arm, Medial cutaneous nerve of forearm, Medial root of median nerve, Ulnar nerve.
"M4U" - Medial pectoral nerve, Medial cutaneous nerve of arm, Medial cutaneous nerve of forearm, Medial root of median nerve, Ulnar nerve
Union of **4 M**edials - Ulnar nerve, **Medial** cutaneous nerve of arm, **Medial** cutaneous nerve of forearm, **Medial** pectoral nerve, **Medial** root of Median Nerve.
5 main nerves of brachial plexus, in order laterally to medially
"My Aunty Rocks My Uncle" - Musculocutaneous, axillary, radial, median, ulnar.

Bowel components
"Dow Jones Industrial Average Closing Stock Report"
From proximal to distal

D	Duodenum
J	Jejunum
I	Ileum
A	Appendix
C	Colon
S	Sigmoid
R	Rectum

Carotid sheath contents

I See 10 CC's in the **IV**

I See	I See (I.C.) = Internal Carotid artery
10	10 = CN **10** (Vagus nerve)
CC	CC = Common Carotid artery
IV	IV = Internal Jugular Vein

Cavernous sinus contents
O TOM CAT
O TOM are lateral wall components, in order from superior to inferior.
CA are the components within the sinus, from medial to lateral. CA
ends at the level of T from O TOM.

O	Occulomotor nerve (III)
T	Trochlear nerve (IV)
O	Ophthalmic nerve (V1)
M	Maxillary nerve (V2)
C	Carotid artery
A	Abducent nerve (VI)
T	T: When written, connects to the T of OTOM

Celiac trunk (Coeliac trunk): branches

Left Hand Side (LHS)

L	Left gastric artery
H	Hepatic artery
S	Splenic artery

Vertebral column

The servant attacks with saw and axe the lumbar, stack and cord

C	Cervical (atlas, axis)
T	Thoracic
L	Lumbar
S	Sacral
C	Coccygeal

Tributaries of the Inferior vena cava

"I Like To Rise So High"

I	Iliac vein (common)
L	Lumbar vein
T	Testicular vein
R	Renal vein
S	Suprarenal vein
H	Hepatic vein

Greater sciatic foramen

Structures passing through greater sciatic foramen below piriformis (S.N.I.P. N.I.P.)

S	Sciatic nerve
N	Nerve to obturator internus
I	Internal pudendal vessel
P	Pudendal nerve
N	Perve to quadratus femoris
I	Inferior gluteal vessels
P	Posterior cutaneous nerve of thigh

Lesser sciatic foramen

Structures passing through lesser sciatic foramen: (P.I.N.T.)

P	Pudendal nerve
I	Internal pudendal vessels
N	Nerve to obturator internus
T	Tendon of obturator internus

Tarsal tunnel

a mnemonic to remember the contents of the Tarsal tunnel from anterior to posterior is "Tom, Dick and Harry" or alternatively "Tom, Dick (and very nervous) Harry" if the artery, vein, and nerve are included.
Subclavian artery
The branches of the subclavian artery can be remembered using **VIT**amin **C** and **D**.

Posterior mediastinum

The contents of posterior mediastinum can be remembered using the mnemonic, "**DATES**"

D	Descending aorta
A	Azygous vein and hemiazygos vein
T	Thoracic duct
E	Esophagus
S	Sympathetic trunk/ganglia.

Superior orbital fissure

Standing room only can be used to remember that

V_1 passes through the Superior orbital fissure
V_2 through the foramen Rotundum
V_3 through the foramen Ovale.

Foramen magnum

Contents of the foramen magnum: **VAMPS-ATM**

V	Vertebral arteries
A	Anterior Spinal artery
M	Meningeal branches of the cervical nerves
P	Posterior spinal arteries
S	Spinal part of the accessory nerve
A	Alar and Apical ligaments of the dense
T	Tectorial membrane
M	Medulla oblongata

Cerebellum

Deep cerebellar nuclei and their positions relative to the midline: "Fat Guys Eat Donuts," where each letter indicates the medial to lateral location in the cerebellar white matter.

F	**nucleus Fastigii**
G	Globose nucleus
E	nucleus Emboliformis
D	Dentate nucleus.

Pes anserinus

A mnemonic to remember the muscles that contribute tendons to the pes anserinus and the innervations of these muscles is **SGT FOT** (SerGeanT FOT)

S	**S- Sartorius**
G	G- Gracilis
T	T- semiTendinosus (from anterior to posterior).
F	F- Femoral nerve
O	O- Obturator nerve
T	T- Tibial division of the sciatic nerve.

Notice the order of the muscles (S, G, T) follows the order of the innervating nerves which correspond to those muscles (F, O, T).

Femoral triangle

The femoral triangle is shaped like the sail of a sailing ship and hence its boundaries can be remembered using the mnemonic, "**SAIL**"

S	Sartorius
A	Adductor longus
IL	Inguinal Ligament.

The order of structures in the femoral triangle is important in the embalming of bodies, as the femoral artery is often exposed and used to pump embalming fluids into the body. The order of this neurovascular bundle can be remembered using the mnemonic, "**NAVY**"

N	Nerve
A	Artery
V	Vein
Y	SEE INSTRUCTIONS BELLOW

Y -fronts (the British term of a style of men's underwear with a "Y" shaped front that acts as a fly). The "Y" is midline (corresponding with the penis) and the mnemonic always reads from lateral to medial (in other words, the Femoral Nerve is always lateral).

An alternate to this mnemonic is "**NAVEL**" for Nerve, Artery, Vein, Empty Space and Lymph, to include the deep inguinal lymph nodes located medial to the Femoral vein.

Popliteal fossa

A useful **mnemonic** to remember popliteal fossa anatomy (medial-to-lateral arrangement) is: Serve And Volley Next Ball.

S	Semimembranosus and semitendinosus (superior medial border)
A	Artery (popliteal artery)
V	Vein (popliteal vein)
N	Nerve (tibial nerve)
B	Biceps femoris (superior lateral border). The lateral and medial heads of gastrocnemius form the inferior border.

Diaphragm apertures: spinal levels

Many mnemonics are used for diaphragm apertures including:
Number of letters

Aortic hiatus = 12 letters = T12
Oesophagus = 10 letters = T10
Vena cava = 8 letters = T8

I ate 10 eggs at 12
I = IVC
ate = T8
10 = T10
Eggs = Esophagus
At = Aorta
12 = T12
 (V)oice (O)f (A)merica
V- vena cava -T8
O-oesophagus-T10
A-aorta-T12

Duodenum: lengths of parts
"Counting 1 to 4 but staggered"
1st part: **2** inches
2nd part: **3** inches
3rd part: **4** inches
4th part: **1** inch
Endocrine glands
The major glands of the endocrine system, excluding ovaries and testes:
"**T-A-P.**" (T2, A3, P4)
Thymus
Thyroid
Anterior pituitary
Adrenal cortex
Adrenal medulla
Posterior pituitary
Parathyroid gland
Pancreas
Pineal

Extraocular muscles
A good mnemonic to remember which muscles are innervated by what nerve is to paraphrase it as a molecular equation: $LR_6SO_4R_3$.
Lateral Rectus - Cranial Nerve **VI**
Superior Oblique - Cranial Nerve **IV**
the **Rest** of the muscles - Cranial Nerve **III**
Another way to remember which nerves innervate which muscles is to understand the meaning behind all the Latin words.
The *fourth cranial nerve*, the trochlear, is so named because the muscle it innervates, the superior oblique, runs through a little fascial pulley that changes its direction of pull (the trochlea of superior oblique). This pulley exists in the superiomedial corner of each orbit, and "trochl-" is Latin for "pulley."
The *sixth cranial nerve*, the *abducens*, is so named because it controls the lateral rectus, which abducts the eye (rotates it laterally) upon contraction.
The *third cranial nerve*, the *oculomotor*, is so named because it is in charge of the movement (motor) of the eye (oculo-). It controls all the other muscles.

G.I. tract layers (simplified)

M.S.M.S

M	Mucosa
S	Submucosa
M	Muscularis propria
S	Serosa

Kidney functions

A WET BED

A	A – maintaining ACID-base balance
W	W – maintaining WATER balance
E	E – ELECTROLYTE balance
T	T – TOXIN removal
B	B – BLOOD Pressure control
E	E – making ERYTHROPOIETIN
D	D – Vitamin D metabolism

Lateral geniculate nucleus

A simple mnemonic for remembering this is "See I? I see, I see," with "see" representing the C in "contralateral," and "I" representing the I in "ipsilateral." Another is "Emily and Pete meet eye to eye" as in "M and P meet I to I," or again, Magno and Parvo meet Ipsi to Ipsi.
Another way of remembering this is 2+3=5, which is correct, so ipsilateral side, and 1+4 doesn't equal 6, so contralateral.

Placenta-crossing substances

WANT My Hot Dog

W	Wastes
A	Antibodies
N	Nutrients
T	Teratogens
M	Microorganisms
H	Hormones, HIV
D	Drugs

Retina

A mnemonic to remember the layers of the retina:

My	Membrane (internal limiting)
Nerves	Nerve fibers
Get	Ganglions
In	Inner plexiform
Knots	Inner nuclear
Outside	Outer plexiform
Our	Outer nuclear
Easy	External limiting membrane
Practice	Photoreceptors
Review	Retinal pigment epithelium

Sperm: path through male reproductive system

"My boyfriend's name is **STEVE**"

S	Seminiferous Tubules
E	Epididymis
V	Vas deferens
E	Ejaculatory duct

Sternal angle
For structures lying at the level of the sternal angle, the following mnemonic can be used:

RAT PLLANT

Rib 2
Aortic arch
Tracheal bifurcation
Pulmonary trunk
Ligamentum arteriosum
Left recurrent laryngeal
Azygos Vein
Nerves (Cardiac and Pulmonary plexuses)
Thoracic duct

PLOT of EARTH PLLANTS
is a more detailed mnemonic including:
Phrenic and Vagus Nerve
Lymph Nodes
Oblique fissure of lungs (top of it)
Thymus
Esophagus (trending right to left)
Aortic Arch (bottom of the arch)
Rib 2, Manubrium-sternal angle, T4(more specifically T4-5 disc)
Tracheal Bifurcation (Carina: Latin –like keel of boat)
Heart
Pulmonary trunk bifurcation
L2 : Left Recurrent Laryngeal (Looping under Aorta); Ligamentum Arteriosum: Connects Aortic Arch to Pulmonary. Bifurcation
Azygous vein arches over the root of the Rt. Lung and opens in SVC.
Nerve plexi: Cardiac and Pulmonary Plexus
Thoracic duct (on its way to drain into the Left Subclavian)
SVC going down

Spine

Breakfast at 7:00--- 7 cervical vertebrae
Lunch at 12:00--- 12 thoracic vertebrae
Dinner at 5:00--- 5 lumbar vertebrae

Hand

Carpal bones:
Some Lovers Try Positions That They Can't Handle:
Scaphoid, Lunatum, Triquetrum, Pisiforme, Trapezium, Trapezoid,
Capitate and Hamate

Carpal Bones:
She Looks Too Pretty Try To Catch Her:
Scaphoid, Lunate, Triquetrum, Pisiforme, Trapezium, Trapezoid,
Capitate and Hamate

Carpal bones:
Scabby Lucy Tried Pissing Hours after Copulating Two Twins:
Scaphoid, Lunate, Triquetrum, Pisiforme, Hamate, Capitate, Trapezoid,
and Trapezium:
In clockwise order from Scaphoid-remember zoids do not touch each
other. M. Hall

Carpal bones:

So Long To Pinky Here Comes The Thumb:
Straight Line To Pinky Here Comes The Thumb:
Scaphoid, Lunatum, Triquetrum, Pisiforme, Hamate, Capitate,
Trapezoid, Trapezium

Internal iliac artery: branches

I Like Going Places Using My Very Own Unmanned Vehicle

Posterior division:
Iliolumbar artery
Lateral sacral artery
Superior gluteal artery
Anterior division:
Inferior gluteal artery
Internal pudendal artery
Umbilical artery
Middle rectal artery
Superior and inferior vesical artery
Obturator artery
Uterine artery (female)
Vaginal artery (female)

Coronal section of brain (structures)

"In Extremis, Cannibals Eat People's Globus Pallidi Instead of Their Hearts":

From insula to midline:
Insula
Extreme capsule
Claustrum
External capsule
Putamen
Globus pallidus
Internal capsule
Thalamus
Hypothalamus

Anterior Pituitary Hormones

FLAG TOP

FSH
LH
ACTH
GH
TSH
MelanOcyte Stimulating Hormone
Prolactin

MISCELLANEOUS

When treating a fracture, keep PRICE in mind.

P	Pressure
R	Rest
I	Ice
C	Compression
E	Elevation

The symptoms of Hyperthyroidism can be grouped as STING.

S	Sweating
T	Tremors or Tachycardia
I	Intolerance to heat, Irregular period, Irritability, Irregular eyes (e.g., weakness or bulging)
N	Nervousness, Neurological (e.g., chorea, myopathy, paralysis)
G	Goitre, Gastrointestinal problems (such as vomiting, nausea, as well as constipation or diarrhea)

ABOUT THE AUTHOR

Maria Youtman MSN BSN RN

Words are very powerful. They can either inspire you to greatness or make you feel like crap. This is why it's best to choose the words you hear and the principles you believe. After all, we are all given a choice ever day: to wallow in self-pity or push ourselves to achieve great things despite our imperfections.

"Maria Youtman, MSN, BSN, RN, earned her bachelor of science degree from Penn University, and her Master of Science in Nursing from Johns Hopkins University. She has 10 years of nursing experience and 6 years of experience as a clinical nurse specialist. For the past Three years, she's overseen nursing care in writing medical articles, books, and more."

Maria had a three years of private clinical education and writing through various websites, she intended to move on one step to have a web community source, whatever she inspired, write, and edit, one place can gather all the efforts made.

Nurses are no exception. One's success in the nursing profession is not determined by how much theoretical knowledge a nurse possesses, but how resilient you are to apply everything you've learned–and that includes the principle of caring.

Nursing is going to become even more important in the coming years. That's because health care systems throughout the world are gradually shifting attention towards models that do more to prevent and manage cardiovascular disease, diabetes and other chronic diseases that are best dealt with in patients before they require hospitalization. Nurses will play an enormous role in these lower-cost, higher-touch, prevent-and-manage models, because the emphasis will be one more frequent bust less intense levels of care that call for coaching, outreach and simple patient self-measurements like blood pressure – routines that often don't require much physician involvement. And as nursing continues to grow higher-level, more specialized branches, the way that physician practice has, nurses will increasingly take over many diagnostic and treatment tasks. It's just one more reason to assign nursing such a high priority."

#Steve Thompson

Made in the USA
Columbia, SC
22 December 2023

29333421R00078